Understanding
THYROID
DISORDERS

Dr Anthony Toft

GW00336488

Published by Family Doctor Publications Limited
in association with the British Medical Association

IMPORTANT

This book is intended to supplement the advice given to you by your doctor. The author and publisher have taken every care in its preparation. In particular, information about drugs and dosages has been thoroughly checked. However, before taking any medication you are strongly advised to read the product information sheet accompanying it. Your pharmacist will be able to help you with anything you do not understand.

© Family Doctor Publications 1995
Reprinted 1996

Medical Editor: Dr Tony Smith
Consultant Editor: Chris McLaughlin
Front Cover Illustration: Colette Blanchard
Medical Artist: Angela Christie
Design: Fox Design, Bramley, Guildford, Surrey
Printing: Cambus Litho, Scotland, using acid-free paper

ISBN: 1 898205 18 3

Contents

Introduction

The thyroid gland lies in front of the neck between the skin and voice box. It has a right and left lobe each about five centimetres in length and joined in the midline. The entire gland weighs less than an ounce (about 20 grams). Despite its small size it is an extremely important organ which controls our metabolism and is responsible for the normal working of every cell in the body. It achieves this by manufacturing the hormones thyroxine (T_4) and triiodothyronine (T_3) and secreting them into the bloodstream. Doctors believe that T_4 only starts to be active when it is converted, mainly in the liver, to T_3.

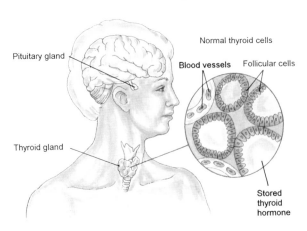

Pituitary gland

Thyroid gland

Normal thyroid cells

Blood vessels   Follicular cells

Stored thyroid hormone

Position and cross-section of normal gland. Normally it cannot be seen or felt.

In healthy people the amounts of T_3 and T_4 in the blood are maintained within narrow limits by a hormone known as thyroid-stimulating hormone (TSH) or thyrotrophin. TSH is secreted by the anterior pituitary gland which is a pea-size structure, hanging from the undersurface of the brain just behind the eyes, and enclosed in a bony depression in the base of the skull. When thyroid disease causes thyroid hormone levels in the blood to fall, TSH secretion from the pituitary is increased; when thyroid hormone levels rise, TSH secretion is switched off – a relationship known as 'negative feedback', familiar to engineers and biologists.

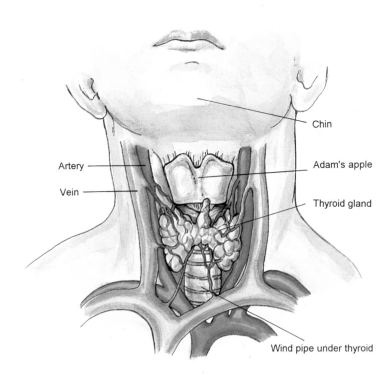

Anatomical view showing thyroid, voice box (larynx), Adam's apple and windpipe (trachea).

If your GP suspects that you may have an underactive thyroid gland (hypothyroidism), his or her diagnosis can be confirmed by sending a sample of your blood to the laboratory for analysis. Low levels of T_3 and T_4 and high levels of TSH in your blood mean that your doctor was right. Similarly, the diagnosis of an overactive thyroid gland (hyperthyroidism) is confirmed by high levels of T_3 and T_4 and low levels of TSH. The results will be available within a few days. Patients with uncomplicated hypothyroidism will not usually be referred to hospital and your GP can prescribe and monitor your treatment. The majority of patients with hyperthyroidism or with abnormal growth of the thyroid gland will be referred to a hospital specialist for further investigation and advice about treatment.

Thyroid disease is common and hyperthyroidism, hypothyroidism or abnormal growth or enlargement of the gland (goitre or thyroid nodule) affects about one in 20 people. Most diseases of the thyroid can be successfully treated, and even thyroid cancer, which is rare, may not lead to a reduction in life expectancy if detected early and appropriately treated.

Thyroid disease often runs in families but in an unpredictable manner and certain forms are associated with an increased risk of developing conditions such as diabetes mellitus or pernicious anaemia. All types of thyroid disease are more common in women.

This following chapters will deal with each of the most common thyroid disorders individually.

KEY POINTS

✓ Thyroid disease is common, affecting around one in 20 people

✓ More women than men are affected

✓ Your GP can diagnose the condition with a simple blood test

✓ Treatment is usually successful, and even thyroid cancer can be cured if caught early

Overactive thyroid

An overactive thyroid (hyperthyroidism or thyrotoxicosis) results from the overproduction of the thyroid hormones, T_4 and T_3, by the thyroid gland. In three-quarters of patients this is due to the presence in the blood of an antibody that stimulates the thyroid not only to secrete excessive amounts of thyroid hormones but also, in some, to increase the size of the thyroid gland, producing a goitre. This type of hyperthyroidism is known as Graves' disease, named after one of the physicians who described the condition in considerable detail over 200 years ago.

The cause of the antibody production is not known but, as Graves' disease runs in families, genes must play a part. There is thought to be some environmental trigger which starts off the disease in genetically susceptible individuals, but the culprit has not been identified. Stress, in the form of major life events, such as divorce or death of a close relative, may play a role.

Some patients with Graves' disease develop prominent eyes (exophthalmos or proptosis) and a few also suffer from raised, red, itchy areas of skin on the front of the lower legs or on the top of the feet, which are known as pretibial myxoedema. These, like the production of the thyroid-stimulating antibodies, are due to an abnormality in the patient's immune system which doctors don't yet fully understand. Most other patients with hyperthyroidism have a goitre containing one or more nodules or 'lumps'. These overproduce thyroid hormones in their own right and are not under the control of TSH, as is the normal thyroid gland.

Graves' disease can come on at any age but most commonly affects women in the 40–50 age group. Hyperthyroidism due to a nodular goitre is unusual before the age of 40.

AN OVERACTIVE THYROID GLAND

In retrospect, most patients will have had symptoms for at least six months before they go to see their doctors, but in some, usually teen-agers, the onset is more rapid with symptoms present for only a few weeks. Not all patients with hyper-thyroidism have all the symptoms listed below. In elderly people the predominant features, in addition to weight loss, are often a reduction in appetite, muscle weakness and apathy. A young woman, on the other hand, may appear to be full of energy and be unable to sit still for more than a few seconds.

Symptoms

● **Weight loss:** This happens to almost all patients due to a 'burning off' of calories caused by the high levels of thyroid hormones in the blood. You will probably find you're hungry all the time, and that you even have to get up in the night to get something to eat. The degree of weight loss varies from 2–3 kilograms to as much as 35 kilo-grams or more but a few people find that their appetite increases to such an extent that they may gain a little weight. If you are severely overweight when the condition first starts, you'll probably

be delighted to find that you're losing weight and put it down to dieting, but sadly you'll put the weight back on once you're being treated.

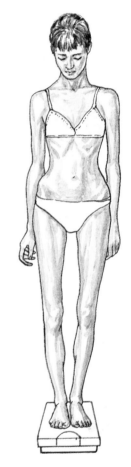

The extent of weight loss is confirmed on the scales. Patients sometimes delay seeing their doctors because they are worried that the weight loss is caused by cancer and do not wish to have their worst fears confirmed.

●**Heat intolerance and sweating:** Because metabolism is increased, your body produces excessive heat which it then gets rid of by sweating. You won't enjoy warm weather or a centrally heated environment and may feel comfortable scantily dressed on a crisp winter's day. In extreme cases, your inability to tolerate heat may lead to disagreements with friends and colleagues as you're constantly turning heating thermostats down, opening windows and tossing blankets or duvet off the bed.

●**Irritability:** This most often affects women with a young family. You may find yourself increasingly unable to cope with the demands and stresses of looking after the children, lose your temper frequently, and find that you're abnormally sensitive to criticism, bursting into tears for no apparent reason. You may find it difficult to concentrate, which can adversely affect your performance at school, college or at work.

●**Palpitations:** Most patients experience palpitations, or you may be aware of your heart beating at a faster rate than normal. In severe, long-standing, untreated hyperthyroidism, particularly in elderly people, there may be an irregular heartbeat, known as atrial fibrillation, and even heart failure.

●**Breathlessness:** This is most likely to be noticeable when you've exerted yourself, for example, after climbing two or three short flights of stairs. Asthmatic individuals may notice a worsening of their symptoms.

●**Tremor:** Most patients complain of shaky hands which may be mistaken by friends and relatives for the tremor of alcoholism. You'll find it difficult to hold a cup still or insert a key into a lock and your handwriting may deteriorate.

●**Muscle weakness:** Characteristically the thigh muscles become weak making it hard to climb stairs or to get up from a squatting position or a low chair without using your arms.

●**Bowel movements:** There tends to be an increase in their frequency such that you pass a softer than normal stool two or three times daily. Diarrhoea can occasionally be a problem.

●**Menstruation:** Periods are often irregular, light or even absent. Until the hyperthyroidism is adequately treated it may be difficult to conceive.

●**Skin, hair and nails:** You may find that your whole body itches, and people with Graves' disease, as

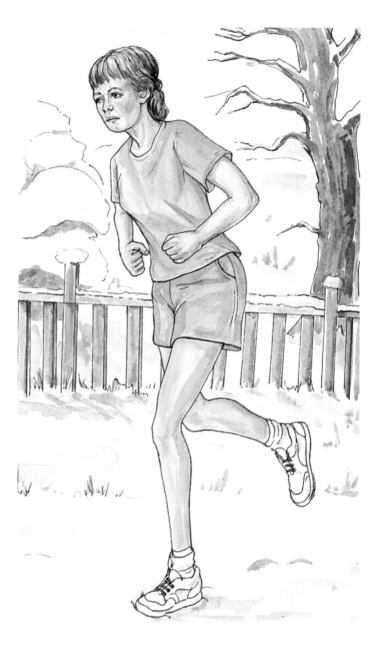

You may feel so warm that you need only tee shirt and shorts even in the snow!

mentioned earlier, may develop raised itchy patches on their lower legs and feet (pretibial myxoedema). Your hair will probably become thinner and finer than usual and won't take a perm very well. Your nails will be brittle and become rather unsightly.

● **Eyes:** It is only those patients with Graves' disease who have trouble with their eyes. These include excessive watering made worse by wind and bright light, pain and grittiness as if there is sand in the eyes, double vision and blurring of vision. Many sufferers are also naturally upset because they develop exophthalmos (protruding eyes) as well as 'bags' under their eyes.

● **Goitre:** Although you will obviously be able to see when you have a goitre, it's unlikely to cause any actual symptoms other than a sensation that there is something in your neck that shouldn't be there.

Confirming the diagnosis

You'll probably have had a blood test taken at your health centre or GP's surgery, but you may well have more done for confirmation when you go to the outpatients' clinic at the hospital. The specialist may also wish to carry out a thyroid scan to obtain more information

about the cause of the hyperthyroidism as this may affect the type of treatment you will need.

A thyroid scan requires a tiny dose of radioactive iodine or technetium to be given either by mouth or by injection into a vein. The dose is so small that it can even be given to someone who is known to be allergic to iodine. Most specialists, however, would try to avoid radioactive scanning if you are pregnant or breast-feeding.

After your GP has made the initial diagnosis, you'll probably have to wait for a bit before you can see the hospital specialist. In the meantime, your symptoms may be eased by taking one of the beta-blocker drugs such as propranolol. This is most likely to be in a dose of 40 milligrams to be taken three or four times daily or in the form of propranolol (Inderal-LA) 160 milligrams daily as a single dose by mouth. Beta-blocking drugs should not be taken by asthmatic individuals.

Treatment for Graves' disease

There are three forms of treatment for the hyperthyroidism due to Graves' disease. These are drugs, surgery and radioactive iodine.

● **Drugs:** Antithyroid drugs are usually given to younger patients who go to their doctor when they

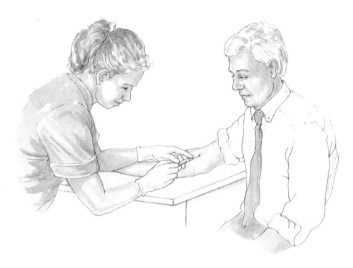

An injection of radioactive technetium is given into a vein and an image of the thyroid is obtained by scanning the neck 20 minutes later.

have their first episode of hyperthyroidism. The most commonly used drug in the UK is carbimazole which reduces the amount of hormones made by the thyroid gland. It is available as 5 milligram and 20 milligram tablets. A high dose (40 to 45 milligrams daily) is used initially and your symptoms should start to improve after 10 to 14 days. Normally treatment is continued for six to 18 months. To start with, your specialist will review your treatment every four to six weeks, and the dose of carbimazole will be reduced in stages down to 5 to 15 milligrams daily in a single dose, depending upon the results of measurements of your blood levels of T_3, T_4 and TSH. Some specialists prefer to give a high dose of

carbimazole throughout treatment, usually as 40 milligrams daily, in the form of two 20-milligram tablets. This would mean you would eventually develop an underactive thyroid gland and therefore thyroxine is added to the carbimazole once thyroid hormone levels have returned to normal. The advantage of this type of treatment is that it doesn't need to be reviewed so often. It can also be particularly beneficial for patients with severe eye disease, but isn't any more effective in controlling symptoms of hyperthyroidism than carbimazole alone.

What you should know: few people will experience any side effects from taking carbimazole, but those who do usually develop them within three to four weeks of starting treatment. A skin rash affects two per cent of patients, but the more serious reaction is a reduction in the number of white blood cells which causes mouth ulcers and infection with a high fever. Your doctor should warn you about these possible effects when you first start the treatment. If you are affected, you should stop taking the drug and contact your GP straight away. You can then be given an alternative drug, called propylthiouracil, which works in a similar way to carbimazole.

● **Surgery:** Unfortunately, despite taking carbimazole or propylthiouracil alone or in combination with thyroxine for up to 18 months, about half of all patients will develop hyperthyroidism again and usually within two years of stopping the drug. If you're under 45 when you have your second bout of the condition, it may be treated surgically by removing about three-quarters of your thyroid gland.

Before this operation can be done, however, it is necessary to restore thyroid hormone levels in your blood to normal with carbimazole. Once you've been given a date for the operation, you may be asked to take an iodine-containing medication for 10 to 14 days before surgery to reduce the size of the thyroid and its blood flow, which makes the job technically simpler for the surgeon. You'll usually go into hospital the day before your operation, which lasts about one hour, and you'll be allowed home between two and four days afterwards.

What you should know: the disadvantage is that you will have a scar, but this usually becomes pale and unnoticeable among the other wrinkles in the neck. Alternatively you can wear jewellery or scarves to hide it. In very rare cases (less than one per cent), the parathyroid glands, which lie close to the thyroid and control the level of calcium in the blood, may be damaged, in which case long-term treatment with vitamin D capsules will be necessary. Equally rare is damage to one of the nerves supplying the voice box which may result in significant alteration to the quality of the voice. Although this wouldn't matter very much to most people, it could make surgery a less acceptable option to anyone who depends upon their voice for a living – an opera singer, for example.

In experienced hands the initial results of surgery are good. Eighty per cent of sufferers will be cured immediately. However, 15 per cent will have had too much thyroid tissue removed and so will be hypothyroid, whereas five per cent will have had insufficient thyroid tissue removed and remain hyper-thyroid. These failures are not due to surgical incompetence but have more to do with the nature of the underlying thyroid disease. What's more, over the passage of time, an increasing proportion of those patients whose hyperthyroidism was originally cured by surgery will develop an underactive thyroid gland. Recurrence of hyperthyroidism may even develop 20 to 40 years after apparently successful surgery.

● **Radioactive iodine (iodine-131):** Traditionally this form of treatment is reserved for patients over 40 to 45 and beyond child-bearing age or for younger individuals who have been sterilized.

This conservative approach was originally adopted because of concern that radioactive iodine might lead to any children conceived after treatment being born with abnormalities. In fact, there is no evidence for this, and in some hospitals there is a move towards using radioactive iodine in younger patients as it is cheap and easy to administer.

Radioactive iodine is taken as a capsule or a drink which tastes like water, and is usually administered in hospital in a department of medical physics. Before receiving treatment you may be asked to sign a consent form, and will have received in-structions about avoiding places of entertainment and close contact with colleagues and young children for a period of a few days after therapy. Radioactive iodine is never prescribed for pregnant women as it will adversely affect the fetal thyroid gland and women are advised to avoid pregnancy for four months following treatment.

The treatment takes six to eight weeks to work and in the interim, depending upon the severity of the hyperthyroidism, you may be given propranolol or carbimazole to relieve your symptoms. You'll be asked to come back to hospital for a check-up in two to three months, and if you're one of the minority of people who is found to be still hyperthyroid, you'll be given a second dose of radioactive iodine.

What you should know: the major problem with this treatment, however, is the development of hypothyroidism. It's most likely to appear in the first year after treatment, affecting about 50 per cent of people in some centres. In each year after that, around two to four per cent of people will be affected. It follows that the great majority become hypothyroid eventually and it is essential that you should have regular check-ups either at the hospital or with your GP. Once hypothyroidism has developed treatment is with thyroxine, ultimately in a dose of 100 to 150 micrograms daily. There are no side effects with thyroxine if the appropriate dose is taken regularly.

CASE 1: JOHN'S STORY

Although 70-year-old John Parry considered himself to be generally very healthy, he had recently noticed that his ankles were swelling. To start with, it was just at night, but then it happened all the time and his legs felt very heavy. One night at 1 a.m. he woke up gasping for breath and coughing up white frothy spit. His wife called an ambulance, and John was admitted to the local hospital within 20 minutes. The doctor on duty, Dr Mackenzie, correctly diagnosed heart failure as the cause of the fluid accumulation in John's legs and lungs. He also noticed that John's pulse rate was very rapid and irregular and an electrocardiogram showed this to be due to atrial fibrillation. Mr Parry was given oxygen using a face mask, an injection of a drug called frusemide (Lasix) to get rid of the excess fluid and digoxin tablets to reduce the speed of his heart beat. Because patients with atrial fibrillation are at risk of throwing off blood clots from the heart resulting in a stroke or a blocked artery in a leg he was also given tablets called warfarin to thin the blood.

WHICH TREATMENT IS RIGHT FOR YOU?

No treatment is perfect and you will need to discuss the options with your specialist. Some patients are not keen on surgery even when a course of antithyroid drugs has been tried and failed.

There is no reason why you shouldn't have a second or even a third course in the hope that the disease will ultimately 'burn itself out'. Indeed before there was any form of treatment for the hyperthyroidism of Graves' disease a proportion of patients got better spontaneously after months or years and then became hypothyroid.

Some patients are unhappy at the prospect of radioactive iodine treatment and some specialists consider that the best treatment for a young patient with severe hyperthyroidism and a large goitre is surgery.

Whatever kind of treatment you have for hyperthyroidism, you will need regular follow-up, usually by an annual blood test taken at a health centre or your GP's surgery.

✓ Around three-quarters of cases of hyperthyroidism are caused by Graves' disease

✓ Many people with Graves' disease may have inherited a tendency to develop it, although other factors are also involved in triggering the condition

✓ The people most likely to develop Graves' disease are women between the ages of 40 and 50

✓ Drugs, surgery and radioactive iodine are all possible ways of treating Graves' disease, but there is no one treatment that is right for everyone

✓ Your specialists may want to discuss the treatment options with you before making the final decision on which approach is best for you

✓ After treatment, you will need regular check-ups to ensure that you stay well

Dr Mackenzie had at one time worked with an eminent endocrinologist and knew that atrial fibrillation could sometimes occur as a complication of an overactive thyroid gland, particularly in older patients.

Mr Parry did indeed have hyperthyroidism which turned out to be due to Graves' disease and he was treated with radioactive iodine. He was also given the antithyroid drug, carbimazole for six weeks until the radioactive iodine had time to take effect.

Although to begin with Mr Parry was concerned about the number of tablets he was taking when he left hospital, these had all been stopped within six months as his thyroid gland came under control. Even his heart is now beating regularly and he is as fit as ever. His GP carries out thyroid blood tests regularly to make sure that Mr Parry is not developing an underactive thyroid gland as a result of the radioactive iodine treatment.

SPECIAL SITUATIONS

Graves' disease in pregnancy

As the thyroid-stimulating antibody responsible for the hyperthyroidism of Graves' disease crosses the placenta and passes from the blood of the mother to that of the developing child, it too will have an overactive thyroid gland like its mother.

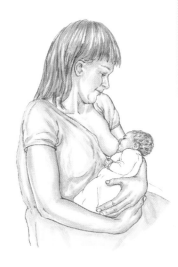

A breast-feeding baby will not be affected by propylthiouracil given to the mother.

Fortunately, the antithyroid drugs also cross the placenta and good control of hyperthyroidism in the mother will ensure that the fetus comes to no harm.

There are some reports from the USA that carbimazole is associated with a rare skin disease, known as aplasia cutis, in the newborn baby. For this reason, a pregnant woman will normally be treated with propylthiouracil. It is available as 50-milligram tablets. She will be prescribed the lowest dose possible to restore the thyroid hormone levels in her blood to normal, and be checked every four to six weeks, in close cooperation with the obstetrician who is caring for her.

The propylthiouracil is usually stopped four weeks before the expected date of delivery. If hyperthyroidism recurs after her baby is born and she is breast-feeding, she will be treated with propylthiouracil rather than carbimazole as it is excreted in the breast milk much less and will not therefore affect the baby.

If you are thinking of trying for a baby, you should tell your doctor and your treatment will be changed to propylthiouracil before you conceive.

CASE 2: FLORA'S STORY

Flora Stewart was 25 and happily married to her lawyer husband, William, and they'd had their first child, Jane, five months earlier. Their relationship began to deteriorate when Flora became weepy and short-tempered, snapping at William for no good reason.

She was also sleeping badly and William noticed that Flora's hands sometimes trembled. However, they both put all this down to hormonal changes following her pregnancy and the birth of their baby, and assumed that before long everything would be back to normal.

However, when Flora began to complain of palpitations William persuaded her to visit their GP.

The doctor thought that Flora might have an overactive thyroid gland and his suspicions were confirmed by a blood test.

On hearing the news Flora was concerned because her mother had suffered from Graves' disease when she was in her thirties and her eyes were still very prominent 20 years later, even though the hyper-thyroidism had been cured. In order to relieve some of Flora's symptoms her GP prescribed a long-acting form of propranolol (Inderal LA) 80 milligrams, to be taken once daily and he suggested that Flora should see a specialist at the local hospital. By the time her appointment came round four weeks later, Flora felt much better and a repeat blood sample showed that her thyroid gland had become very slightly underactive. The diagnosis was not that of Graves' disease, but postpartum thyroiditis, and Flora was reassured that she would not get bulging eyes like her mother. The propranolol was stopped, and another blood test two months later was entirely normal.

Flora now knows that she may get the symptoms of postpartum thyroiditis following further pregnancies, and that she has an increased chance of developing a permanently underactive thyroid gland at some stage in the future.

However, her GP will do a thyroid blood test every year to make sure that it is detected before she can develop severe symptoms.

CASE 3: ANNA'S STORY

Anna Robinson had had a previous episode of hyperthyroidism caused by Graves' disease in her mid-twenties, for which she had been given an 18-month course of carbimazole. At the age of 45, she noticed that she was troubled by the heat, but put this symptom down to the 'change of life'.

However, when she began to lose weight and her hands became shaky, she realized that her thyroid gland was overactive again. At the local hospital the specialist suggested that she should be treated with radioactive iodine. In spite of reassurances and the evidence that this form of treatment was not associated with any risk other than the eventual onset of an underactive thyroid gland, Mrs Robinson was uneasy. She was aware of articles in the newspapers of a possible link between radiation and leukaemia in those living near to nuclear power stations, and she did not like the thought of avoiding her new grand-daughter albeit only for a few days after treatment.

As she was a keen singer in the local church choir, thyroid surgery was felt not to be appropriate because of the possibility of a change in the quality of her voice.

Mrs Robinson was relieved to learn that there was no reason why she could not be treated with carbimazole now or in the future.

Graves' disease and the eyes

Most patients with Graves' disease will show signs of eye disease (ophthalmopathy) if the doctor looks hard enough. Sometimes the eye disease may occur before the onset of the overactive thyroid gland and even for the first time many years after the successful treatment of the hyperthyroidism. Treatment of the eye disease is not as satisfactory as that of the overactive thyroid gland. Smoking is thought to make it worse as does poor control of the hyperthyroidism. It is very important, therefore, that you stop smoking completely and are careful to follow your doctor's instructions about dosage of tablets such as carbimazole or thyroxine. If you suffer from excessive watering, you may find that a prescription for artificial tears helps, and it's worth wearing dark glasses when sunny.

Those with more advanced disease due to a build-up of pressure behind the eye which threatens vision may need treatment with a steroid drug such as prednisolone. Alternatively, an operation may be required to remove part of the wall of the bony cavity (the orbit) in which the eye sits. Such a major undertaking is rarely necessary, however, and would only be carried out after close collaboration between thyroid and eye specialists. Most people with Graves' disease find that their eye problems settle down considerably over a period of two to three years. At that stage relatively minor surgery will correct double vision and reduce the 'staring' look and the bags under the eyes.

There is some evidence to suggest that the eye disease may deteriorate after treatment with radioactive iodine and some specialists will not wish to prescribe this form of therapy for anyone whose eyes are badly affected.

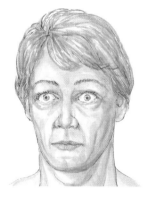

Prominence of the eyes often alerts the patient or her relatives to the possibility of an overactive thyroid gland.

Nodular goitre

This is treated either with surgery or with radioactive iodine. Unlike someone with Graves' disease, you're unlikely to develop hypothyroidism. It used to be fashionable after surgery to prescribe thyroxine to prevent regrowth of the goitre, but this is not really useful unless you've developed hypothyroidism.

RARER TYPES OF HYPERTHYROIDISM

- Some women may develop mild hyperthyroidism, lasting for a few weeks, in the first year after the birth of a baby. Some then also experience a short period of mild hypo-thyroidism. This condition is known as postpartum thyroiditis and may occur following further pregnancies. It rarely needs any treatment other than a beta-blocking drug, such as propranolol.

- A similar disturbance of thyroid function may occur after a viral infection of the thyroid; this is known as viral or de Quervain's thyroiditis and the most prominent feature is severe pain and tenderness over the thyroid gland associated with symptoms of a 'flu-like illness.

- The iodine-containing drug, amiodarone, which is used increasingly by heart specialists for the treatment of certain irregularities of heart rhythm, may cause hyperthyroidism. Your blood thyroid levels should be checked before you start taking the drug, and at six-monthly intervals while you're on it.

KEY POINTS

✓ If you are planning a baby, tell your doctor as you may need to take a different drug from your usual one

✓ Your doctors will keep a close watch on you during pregnancy, but your treatment will not harm your developing baby

✓ Most people with Graves' disease will experience some degree of eye problems, although they may only be minor irritations. More serious symptoms can be treated and usually settle in time

✓ Some women will develop mild thyroid disease after having a baby, but this is easily treated. If you are experiencing similar symptoms to those described in Flora's story on page 15, it is worth asking your GP whether this could be the cause

Underactive thyroid

An underactive thyroid (hypothyroidism) occurs when the thyroid gland stops producing enough of the thyroid hormones, T_3 and T_4. In its most common form, affecting one per cent of the population, mainly middle-aged and elderly women, the thyroid gland shrinks as its cells are all destroyed by a subtle defect in the patient's immune system. Less often this defect leads not only to hypothyroidism but to thyroid enlargement and the formation of a goitre. This is known as Hashimoto's thyroiditis. These types of hypothyroidism are associated, as is Graves' disease, with the other so-called 'autoimmune diseases' shown in the box.

Although having hypothyroidism makes you more likely to develop one or more of these conditions than other people, the risk is still small. The other reason why people develop hypothyroidism is as a result of treatment of Graves' disease by surgery or with radioactive iodine.

AN UNDERACTIVE THYROID GLAND

Hypothyroidism does not come on overnight but slowly over many months and you and your family may not notice the symptoms at first, or may simply put them down to ageing.

GPs now have ready access to the appropriate laboratory tests and, as a result, hypothyroidism is increasingly likely to be diagnosed at a relatively early stage when symptoms are mild. Hypothyroidism in its advanced state is sometimes known as 'myxoedema'.

It would be unusual to have all the symptoms mentioned below unless the diagnosis had been delayed for some reason for months or even years. You're more likely to go to your GP with rather vague

- Pernicious anaemia for which regular injections of vitamin B_{12} are necessary to maintain a normal blood count.

- Diabetes mellitus usually requiring treatment with insulin.

- Addison's disease: the adrenal glands which sit on top of each kidney produce insufficient cortisol and aldoster-one, hormones that fortunately can be taken as tablets.

- Premature ovarian failure which causes loss of periods, infertility and an early menopause.

- Underactivity of the glands adjacent to the thyroid, the parathyroid glands, leads to a low level of calcium in the blood and tetany which is effectively treated with vitamin D capsules.

- Vitiligo, a skin disease in which there are areas of loss of pigmentations, gives a 'piebald' appearance.

complaints such as tiredness and weight gain, which could be due to a variety of causes.

You'll have a blood test and, if the result shows you have low T_4 and high TSH levels, this will be confirmation that you are suffering from hypothyroidism. Unless there is a complication, such as angina, you will be treated by your family doctor.

Symptoms

- **Weight gain:** Most patients gain from 5 to 10 kilograms, although your appetite is normal or even less than usual.

- **Sensitivity to the cold:** You'll feel the cold very badly, and want to wear extra layers of clothing and sit close to the fire. You may well suffer from muscle stiffness and spasm when you move suddenly, especially when it's cold.

- **Mental problems:** Tiredness, sleepiness and slowing down intellectually. Your reactions get slow, but fortunately, your sense of humour is unaffected. Older patients may be wrongly thought to be suffering from dementia, while some people experience depression and paranoia, which are the basis

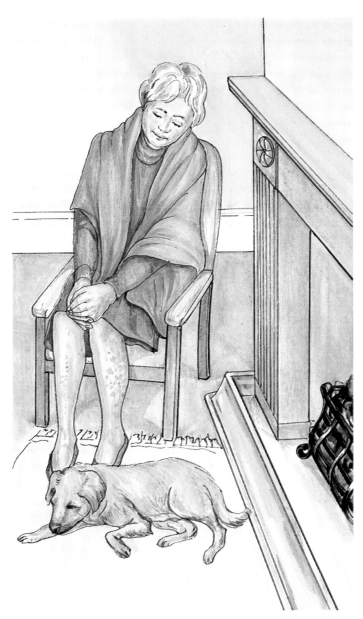

You may still feel cold, even sitting right in front of the fire. If you sit too close for too long your legs will become mottled.

for what is popularly known as 'myxoedema madness'.

●**Speech:** your voice becomes slow and husky and speech is often slurred.

●**Heart:** in contrast to a person with an overactive thyroid gland, your pulse rate is slow at around 60 beats per minute. You may have high blood pressure and an elderly patient with severe long-standing hypothyroidism is at risk of heart failure. Angina may the first symptom of hypothyroidism.

●**Bowel movements:** You probably suffer from constipation.

●**Menstruation:** Your periods become heavier (menorrhagia) if you haven't yet had your menopause.

●**Skin and hair:** Your skin is likely to be rough and dry and to flake readily. It tends to be pale and your eyelids, hands and feet swell. Some people may find their skin has a lemon-yellowish tint and prominent blood vessels in the cheeks add a purplish flush. Sitting too close to the fire can cause a 'granny's tartan' to appear on the skin of your legs. A lot of people get the skin condition known as vitiligo. Your hair becomes dry and brittle and the outer part of your eyebrows may be missing.

●**Nervous system:** You may become a little deaf and have trouble with your balance. If your fingers tingle, especially during the night, shaking your hands vigorously should relieve it.

Treatment

This is with thyroxine which is available in the United Kingdom as 25, 50 and 100-microgram tablets. Normally, thyroxine treatment is begun slowly and you'll be prescribed a daily dose of 50 micrograms for three to four weeks, increasing to 100 micrograms daily for a further three to four weeks and then to 150 micrograms daily. You'll then have another blood test some three months after starting treatment to assess whether any further minor adjustment of dose is necessary. The aim is to restore levels of T_4 and TSH in the blood to normal.

You should start to feel better within two to three weeks; you'll lose weight and notice the puffiness around your eyes disappearing quite soon, but your skin and hair texture may take three to six months to recover fully. Normally you'll have to expect to stay on thyroxine treatment for life.

CASE 4: JEAN'S STORY

Jean Spencer was 17 and in her final year at school, hoping to go to university to study law. She had had diabetes since she was 11 and gave herself insulin injections twice each day. Control of her diabetes had always been very satisfactory and her dose of insulin did not vary much. She had been puzzled, however, for the last three months because she did not seem to require as much insulin as before. On four occasions she had almost become unconscious in class because of a low level of glucose in her blood but had been brought round with sugary drinks by her teacher.

Once she did not respond and was rushed to hospital and given a glucose drip into a vein and kept in overnight. Jean's parents and her teacher were also concerned because she was not concentrating in class and her results in the mock exams had not been nearly as good as expected. She had also begun to complain of the cold and had not been able to sing in the school Christmas Concert because her voice had become husky. It was her aunt, visiting from Canada, who recognized the change in Jean's appearance since her last visit the previous year. She herself had developed an underactive thyroid gland 10 years earlier and suggested to Jean that she have a blood test. Jean is now taking thyroxine tablets, like her aunt, and her insulin dose has returned to its previous level. She passed her A levels with flying colours and is now in her first term at university studying law.

KEY POINTS

✓ Hypothyroidism usually comes on slowly and your symptoms are likely to be vague at first

✓ Your GP will be able to confirm the diagnosis with a simple blood test

✓ Treatment is with tablets, which you'll probably need to take for the rest of your life

SPECIAL SITUATIONS
Pregnancy

The dose of thyroxine may need to be increased during pregnancy by as much as 50 micrograms daily. Blood tests will be taken every three months to check whether the dose needs to be increased. The fetus' thyroid gland develops independently of the mother and makes its own thyroid hormones. Your baby won't be at risk if you forget the occasional dose of thyroxine but if you make a habit of not taking it, you face a bigger chance of having a miscarriage. Very occasionally a baby born to a mother with an underactive thyroid gland will develop hypothyroidism shortly after birth. This will be detected by the National Screening Programme for congenital hypothyroidism and,

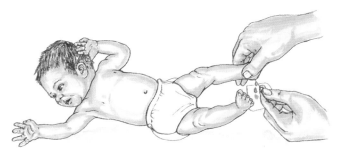

A blood sample is taken from the heel of a newborn baby a few days after birth.

if treatment is necessary, there will be no long-term harm to the child.

Congenital hypothyroidism

One in approximately every 3,500 newborn babies has an underactive thyroid gland. In the past, the problem was not recognized until the child was several weeks old, by which time he or she would be likely to suffer mental and physical retardation. Today, however, all newborn babies are screened by a blood test for the presence of hypothyroidism between five and seven days after they're born. Any affected children are given prompt treatment which ensures that they develop normally.

Angina

The level of various fats or lipids in the blood is increased in hypothyroidism and in people who've had the condition for a long time, the coronary arteries become narrowed by fatty deposits. Insufficient blood reaches the heart muscle, especially during exercise, and the sufferer will get pain in the middle of their chest (angina).

Treatment with thyroxine may worsen the angina and someone with this problem will be started on a lower dose and have it increased more slowly than normal. It may be necessary to have an operation to improve the blood flow through the coronary arteries before or after starting thyroxine treatment.

TEMPORARY HYPOTHYROIDISM

Treatment with thyroxine is usually for life. However, if you develop hypothyroidism in the first three to four months after surgery or radioactive iodine treatment for Graves' disease it may be short-lived, lasting only a few weeks, and you may not need any treatment. The same is true for the hypothyroidism which is a complication of postpartum thyroiditis or de Quervain's thyroiditis (see page 18).

MILD HYPOTHYROIDISM

Most GPs will arrange for someone to have a blood test even when they only suspect thyroid problems, so quite minor abnormalities are often picked up in patients who come because of a variety of rather vague symptoms, such as tiredness, or in people who have a family history of autoimmune disease. The most common finding is the combination of a 'normal' T_4 but raised TSH level, known among doctors as subclinical hypothyroidism. It is known that around five to 20 per cent of these people will develop more obvious hypothyroidism in each following year. For this reason, it is now common practice to 'nip things in the bud' by prescribing thyroxine when the abnormality has been found on more than one occasion. This may not have any dramatic effect on the individual concerned, but preventive medicine is better than cure.

HYPOTHYROIDISM CAUSED BY DRUGS

One drug, called lithium carbonate, which is widely used for depression and mania, may cause goitre and hypothyroidism. When, as normally happens, a person needs to keep taking lithium carbonate, continued treatment with thyroxine will be necessary.

Amiodarone, used in the treatment of certain heart irregularities, may not only cause hyperthyroidism but also hypothyroidism and anyone who is taking it will need thyroid blood tests from time to time.

KEY POINTS

✓ Although your child may be born with hypothyroidism if you suffer from it, like all newborns he or she will be given a routine test shortly after birth and treated if necessary

✓ Some people who've been hypothyroid for many years may suffer from chest pain caused by angina, and because thyroxine aggravates the problem, their dosage will need careful monitoring. If you already have angina when your thyroid condition is first discovered, your treatment will be adjusted to take account of this

✓ If your thyroid blood test is only slightly abnormal, you may be given preventive treatment with thyroxine

Enlarged thyroid

An enlarged thyroid gland is known as a goitre. There are many causes including a shortage of iodine in the diet which occurs in remote mountainous parts of the world, drugs such as lithium carbonate (Priadel), and autoimmune disorders such as Hashimoto's thyroiditis (see page 19) and Graves' disease (see pages 14–17). The cause of most goitres in this country is not known, however. Such goitres are called 'simple goitres' despite the fact that there are almost certainly complex reasons for their development. Although the thyroid gland is enlarged it continues to produce normal amounts of hormones and the patient is referred to as 'euthyroid' as opposed to hyperthyroid or hypothyroid. At first, in teenagers and young adults, the goitre is evenly or diffusely enlarged. During the next 15 to 25 years whatever caused the thyroid to grow abnormally in the first place remains and it continues to grow but becomes full of lumps or nodules. By the time the young person reaches middle age, the goitre will have become lumpy, when it is known medically as a 'multinodular goitre'.

SIMPLE DIFFUSE GOITRE

Most of those who have a diffuse simple goitre are young women between the ages of 15 and 25. If you are one of them, you (or your relatives) will have noticed a symmetrical, smooth swelling in the front of your neck. You may have had it for some years but thought it was just 'puppy fat'. The goitre will move up and down when you swallow. It is not tender, however, and does not usually cause difficulty in swallowing but you may experience a tight sensation in your neck. The goitre may vary slightly in size and be more noticeable at the time of a period or during pregnancy. It isn't normally a problem appearance-wise – quite the opposite as far as some people are concerned. For example, the great seventeenth and eighteenth century artists often added a goitre to the female figure to enhance her beauty!

Confirming the diagnosis
Usually your GP will want you to be seen by a specialist to exclude the rarer causes of goitre. He can normally do this by feeling your neck and by taking blood tests.

Treatment
No treatment is necessary. In the past iodine (often added to milk) or thyroxine tablets were given but neither is effective. Many people find that their goitre becomes less noticeable or even disappears over a period of two to three years.

SIMPLE MULTINODULAR GOITRE
If you are middle-aged, you will probably become aware of a swelling in your neck while washing or applying make-up in front of a mirror. In fact, the goitre will have been present for many years but has now reached a critical size or it may be that your neck has become thinner. The goitre is often more obvious on one side of the neck than the other. It may vary in size from being barely visible to other

people to so large that you feel you have to hide it by wearing scarves or high-necked sweaters. A few people notice the enlarged thyroid gland for the first time because internal bleeding causes increased swelling which is accompanied by discomfort in the neck, like a bruise, lasting a few days. If the goitre is large there may be difficulty in swallowing dry, solid food and, if the trachea (windpipe) is squashed to any extent there may be difficulty in breathing and singers, in particular, will notice a change in their voice.

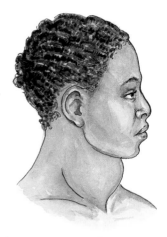

Young woman with a swelling in her neck.

Confirming the diagnosis
Your GP may take a blood sample to check that your thyroid hormone levels are normal but will usually ask a specialist for advice about further investigations and treatment.

The specialist may wish to carry out one or more of the following tests.

● **X-ray and breathing tests:** These will reveal whether the goitre is compressing or squashing the windpipe.

● **Ultrasound scan:** A probe, the size of a small hand torch, is passed

which shows whether the nodules in the goitre are likely to be producing thyroid hormones. It is obtained by injecting a tiny amount of radioactivity in the form of a radioactive substance called tech-netium-99m into a vein. About half an hour after the injection you lie under a sophisticated form of camera for a few minutes.

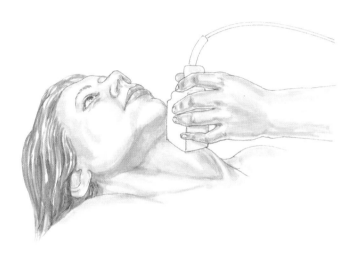

Ultrasound scanning of the thyroid.

over the skin of the front of the neck and an image of the goitre is formed on a TV screen. As well as showing its size and extent it will also highlight any cysts or nodules which the specialist may not have noticed by examining the neck.

● **Isotope scan:** This technique provides a different type of image

● **Fine needle aspiration:** This involves attaching a needle of the same size as that used for taking a blood sample to the end of a syringe, then, while you're lying down, passing it without local anaesthetic through the skin of the neck into the enlarged thyroid gland. By pulling on the plunger and moving the needle up and down a tiny distance within the goitre, the doctor can obtain thyroid cells for analysis. These are smeared on to a glass slide and, after processing in the pathology laboratory, are examined under a microscope. The appearance of the cells will help to determine whether the thyroid enlargement is due to a malignant tumour. Fine needle aspiration, commonly known as FNA, is not often carried out in patients with a multinodular goitre unless the gland is very much bigger on one side than the other, or the goitre is growing very rapidly.

Treatment

If your goitre is relatively small, you probably won't need any treatment. Your GP will check thyroid hormone levels in your blood every one to two years as there is a possibility of the gland becoming overactive and causing hyperthyroidism at some stage during the next 20 years or so. Although thyroxine tablets are prescribed in certain parts of the world in an attempt to shrink the goitre they are of little or no benefit and may cause hyperthyroidism.

If the goitre becomes so large that it looks really unattractive or is compressing the windpipe the most effective treatment is an operation to remove most of the thyroid gland. No treatment is necessary before surgery and you'll be in hospital for about three days. The complications are the same as those for surgery for Graves' disease (page 11). You may have to take

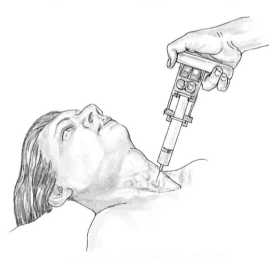

Aspiration of a lump in the neck.

thyroxine treatment afterwards as there may be insufficient thyroid tissue left to produce adequate amounts of hormones.

In patients who aren't fit enough for surgery or who don't want to have an operation, it may be possible to reduce the size of the goitre by about 50 per cent by giving radioactive iodine. A large dose is necessary, and you may have to be admitted to hospital for two or three days. If so, you'll be given a single room to avoid contaminating other patients and visitors with radioactivity. It may take several months for the goitre to shrink. It is unlikely that the thyroid will become underactive.

CASE 5: JENNY'S STORY

Jenny Morris was a single woman in her seventies who had been an accomplished actress. She always wore a silk scarf around her neck, day and night, summer and winter. Friends and neighbours thought it was part of her slightly eccentric personality, but when she was admitted to hospital as an emergency with abdominal pain due to gallstones the scarf was removed to reveal a large goitre and a scar from a previous thyroid operation.

Miss Morris explained that the operation had been carried out for a goitre when she was quite young. In her mid-forties the goitre appeared again but she was told

KEY POINTS

- ✓ In this country, the cause of a goitre usually remains a mystery

- ✓ Young people with a simple diffuse goitre rarely need any treatment

- ✓ You'll probably be referred to a specialist to have a multinodular goitre investigated, and may have several tests

- ✓ A small goitre may be left alone, but you'll have regular blood tests done by your GP as there's a chance of developing hyperthyroidism later on

- ✓ An operation or treatment with radioactive iodine may be necessary if the goitre is causing problems

- ✓ Thyroxine tablets won't help to shrink a goitre, although they are still prescribed in some other countries

further surgery was out of the question because a second operation was technically more difficult and any damage to the nearby nerve supply to the voice box (larynx) would ruin her stage career. As time passed the goitre gradually grew and grew, and she took to wearing the scarves to avoid embarrassment.

Blood tests in hospital showed her to have a slightly overactive thyroid gland and three months after treatment with radioactive iodine her blood test came back normal. Equally important, a year later, the size of the goitre had been reduced by at least a half, and she happily abandoned her scarves!

THYROID NODULES

Single lumps or nodules in the thyroid are common, and can occur at any age. Women are more likely to be affected than men.

OUTCOME OF FNA

- The needle will remove fluid and the nodule will disappear: this means that the nodule must have been a thyroid cyst and no further treatment is needed. Should the cyst recur it can be aspirated again but if it comes back yet again, you will need an operation to remove that half of the thyroid containing the cyst.

- The cells removed from the nodule show that it is a benign lump and therefore you don't have cancer. Unless the swelling is sufficiently large to be disfiguring, when surgery would be necessary, you can be reassured that no treatment is needed.

- The cells removed are malignant which means that the nodule is thyroid cancer, and you will need an immediate operation.

- Sometimes, because of the small number of cells removed, it may be impossible to be certain whether the nodule is benign or malignant (cancer). In this case, you will need an operation to remove the entire nodule so that it can be examined carefully under the microscope.

A single thyroid nodule

The nodule varies in size from that of a pea to a golf ball or even larger. Like a goitre, the nodule is usually discovered by accident while you're washing or looking in a mirror. Bleeding into the nodule may cause pain which alerts you to its presence. Alternatively, the nodule may be discovered during medical examination for some quite unrelated problem, although neither you nor your family had noticed it before. Most women are aware of the significance of a lump in the breast, and so naturally suspect that a nodule in the thyroid may also mean cancer.

This is why your GP will probably want you to see a specialist. In fact, the great majority of single thyroid nodules are not cancers of the thyroid.

Confirming the diagnosis

If you have a single thyroid nodule, your blood test will show normal levels of T_3, T_4 and TSH, which means you're classified medically as 'euthyroid'; the exception is the 'toxic adenoma' in which the thyroid blood tests will demonstrate an overactive thyroid gland. The thyroid specialist will wish to examine your neck carefully as about half of all patients thought to have a single nodule are in fact found to have generalized nodular enlargement of the thyroid known

as multinodular goitre. In this case you can be assured that your condition is not serious.

Those people who need further investigations may have an X-ray, ultrasound or radioisotope scan of their thyroid, but the single most important test is fine needle aspiration (FNA) of the lump.

The technique is simple, quick and, if necessary, can be carried out two or three times as it doesn't cause pain or undue discomfort. FNA is one of the most important advances in the caring for people with thyroid disease. In the past the majority of those with a single thyroid nodule had to have surgery but many operations can now be avoided simply by examining a small sample of thyroid cells obtained by aspiration in the out-patient clinic. The outcome will be one of those indicated in the box.

Benign (non-cancerous) nodules may continue to enlarge over many years and eventually may get so big that an operation is needed to remove them for the sake of your appearance.

If you can't help worrying about the possibility that the lump is harbouring a cancer, your specialist may well suggest operating to remove the nodule so that it can be examined microscopically and resolve the question once and for all.

✓ Although people who develop thyroid nodules often worry that the lump may be cancer, this rarely turns out to be the case

✓ A thyroid blood test will usually reveal normal hormone levels

✓ The simple and painless investigation known as fine needle aspiration means that far fewer people now have to have surgery

✓ If you're concerned about your appearance or can't stop worrying about the possibility of cancer, you can have an operation to remove the nodule

Thyroid cancer

Malignant tumours of the thyroid gland are rare. For example, a specialist may see 50 to 100 patients with hyperthyroidism due to Graves' disease for every one with thyroid cancer. The types which doctors see most frequently are:

- Papillary cancer which affects children and young women.
- Follicular cancer which is unusual before the age of 30.

Both cancers can occur at any age, however. Provided diagnosis and treatment are at an early stage, the person may well live out a normal lifespan; in other words, you're still more likely to die of a stroke or a heart attack in old age.

CONFIRMING
THE DIAGNOSIS

Most patients visit their GP with a lump in the neck or because of rapid growth of a goitre which they've had for many years. The diagnosis of thyroid cancer is made at a hospital visit by fine needle aspiration or following surgery.

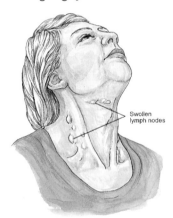

Swollen
lymph nodes

Position of swollen lymph nodes. In some cases the thyroid cancer may not be visible even though the lymph nodes are enlarged.

Occasionally, the patient consults their doctor because of enlarged lymph nodes in the neck which may at first be thought to be caused by Hodgkin's disease. However, a biopsy shows that the patient actually has papillary cancer which has spread from the thyroid gland via the lymphatic system to the nearby lymph nodes.

TREATMENT
Surgery
Papillary cancer is usually treated by removal of as much of the thyroid gland as possible (total thyroidectomy) because there is a tendency for the cancer to occur in various places throughout the gland. Any large lymph nodes containing the cancer are also removed at this stage. In contrast, follicular cancer usually develops in only one part of the thyroid and removal of half of the gland (hemithyroidectomy) is all that may be necessary.

No special treatment is required before the operation and you can usually go home after three days.

Radioactive iodine
It is not possible to remove every last part of the thyroid gland by means of surgery and some patients with papillary cancer will be given a large dose of radioactive iodine (iodine-131) to kill any remaining cells. The radioactive iodine is given as a liquid or a capsule in hospital. You will have to stay in hospital for three to four days, in a single room,

separated from the other patients.

The radioactive iodine is usually given three to four weeks after your operation and before thyroxine tablets have been started as it is most effective when the patient is hypothyroid and TSH levels in the blood are high. If for some reason there is a delay and you have already started taking thyroxine to prevent you from becoming hypothyroid after removal of your thyroid gland, you will be taken off the treatment some four weeks before being given the radioactive iodine.

Towards the end of the period without thyroxine you may feel tired but will come to no harm.

Radioactive iodine is not given so often postoperatively to patients with a follicular cancer.

Thyroxine
Doctors believe that the rate of growth of papillary and follicular cancers of the thyroid may be increased by the hormone TSH. An important part of the treatment, therefore, is to make sure that you take enough thyroxine to ensure that the level of TSH in your blood becomes undetectable.

Patients with thyroid cancer need a slightly greater dose of thyroxine than those with hypothyroidism. A dose of 150 to 200 micrograms daily is usually sufficient to switch off TSH secretion by the pituitary gland.

FOLLOW-UP

Papillary and follicular cancers, like the normal thyroid gland, make a substance called thyroglobulin.

The thyroid gland can only secrete this substance in the presence of TSH, but this is not the case with thyroid cancer. So, if there is no TSH detectable in the bloodstream because it has been suppressed by treatment with thyroxine, any thyroglobulin in the blood must be coming from recurrent cancer in the neck or from cancer that has spread to other parts of the body (secondaries or metastases).

Thyroglobulin is known as a 'tumour marker'. If a patient who is taking appropriate amounts of thyroxine has a raised level of thyroglobulin, the specialist may wish to perform a scan of the whole body using radioactive iodine to identify the site of the recurrent tumour or its metastases.

The scan is usually performed 24 to 48 hours after a dose of iodine-131 by mouth, four weeks after the patient has stopped taking thyroxine. Any tumour that is found may be treated with a large dose of radioactive iodine in hospital.

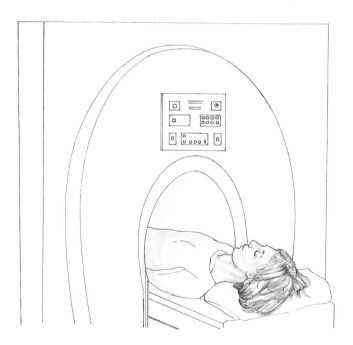

Scanning of the entire body to find out if the cancer has spread beyond the thyroid gland.

OUTLOOK

This depends upon the size of the tumour and whether it has spread at the time of diagnosis. If treated correctly, a young woman with a small papillary cancer of the thyroid is likely to have a normal life expectancy, despite the cancer having spread to the lymph nodes in the neck. Even patients with follicular cancer that has spread to the bones or lung may survive for many years with a good quality of life.

CASE 6: SUSAN'S STORY

Susan Jones was 18 when she fell heavily while skating, striking the side of her neck against the ice-rink barrier. As the pain and bruising settled she noticed a pea-sized lump in her neck. To begin with her doctor thought that it must be related to the accident, although it moved when she swallowed, suggesting that it lay within the thyroid gland rather than in skin or muscle.

When it hadn't disappeared after six weeks, he referred Susan to a thyroid specialist at the local teaching hospital. The consultant examined Susan's neck carefully and found that, in addition to the single small thyroid nodule, there were three enlarged lymph nodes on the right side of her neck. He proceeded to take a tiny sample from the thyroid nodule and from one of the lymph nodes, sucking out cells with a syringe and needle. The test took only a few minutes, causing Susan no discomfort and with no need even for a local anaesthetic.

The next day Susan and her mother were informed that the sample had shown that the lump in Susan's neck was a type of cancer of the thyroid, known as papillary carcinoma, and that it had spread to the nearby lymph nodes. The only treatment was an operation and two weeks later Susan was admitted to hospital where almost all of her thyroid gland was removed, together with the enlarged lymph nodes. Careful inspection of the removed gland by the pathologists showed no other signs of thyroid cancer apart from the original swelling.

Susan has been cured and simply needs to take thyroxine tablets for the rest of her life and see the specialist every year for a blood test. The skating accident was a blessing in disguise as it brought to light a thyroid cancer which was at a very early stage. The fact that it had spread to the lymph nodes in the neck was of no consequence.

RARER CANCERS

These include the following:

● Medullary cancer of the thyroid which can occur on its own or may run in families in association with abnormalities of other endocrine glands or of the skeleton.

- Lymphoma of the thyroid which usually affects elderly people and may be accompanied by evidence of disease in other parts of the body.

- Anaplastic cancer which also affects elderly people.

The future prospects for people with these types of thyroid cancer is less good than for those with papillary or follicular cancer and the treatment is more difficult.

KEY POINTS

✓ Remember that thyroid cancer is rare

✓ The two types which doctors most often see – papillary and follicular cancers – can normally be treated successfully if they are caught early enough

✓ Depending on the type, an operation is necessary to remove all or part of the thyroid gland, and those with papillary cancer may then need treatment with radioactive iodine to destroy any remaining cells

✓ After surgery, patients will need to take thyroxine in slightly higher doses than normal

✓ A blood test will probably be done after treatment to make sure that there is no trace of cancer remaining and to check that it hasn't spread

✓ There are a few very rare cancers which mainly affect elderly people in whom treatment may be more difficult

●**Do I have to change my diet?**
You may have heard that iodine has something to do with the thyroid gland. Indeed iodine is an integral part of the thyroxine (T_4) and triiodothyronine (T_3) molecules. A lack of iodine in the diet may cause a goitre or even hypothyroidism. This is commonly found in people who live in mountainous areas far from the sea such as the Himalayas, but the diet in the UK contains adequate amounts of iodine and you don't need to take supplements. For the disbelievers iodized salt is available in some supermarkets. Excessive iodine intake, however, may unmask underlying thyroid disease and cause both hyperthyroidism and hypothyroidism.

●**Is smoking harmful?**
The eye disease which accompanies Graves' disease is more common and more severe among patients who smoke. Patients with hyperthyroidism due to Graves' disease should stop smoking.

●**Was stress responsible for making my thyroid gland over-active?**
Although it is difficult to prove, most thyroid specialists are impressed by how often major life events, such as divorce or death of a close relative, appear to have taken place a few months before the onset of hyperthyroidism due to Graves' disease. There is now evidence that stress can affect the immune system which is abnormal in Graves' disease. So the answer is probably 'yes' but there are other important factors such as heredity.

●**Will my new baby have thyroid trouble?**
The children of mothers with Graves' disease or a previous

history of Graves' disease may be born with an overactive thyroid gland. This is known as neonatal thyrotoxicosis and lasts for only a few weeks. The obstetrician and the paediatrician will be looking out for this rare complication which is readily treated. Occasionally mothers with hypothyroidism give birth to a child with an underactive thyroid gland. Again this is usually shortlived and will be detected by the routine blood testing of all babies a few days after birth.

● Will my children be affected?

Not necessarily. In fact, the risk is relatively small, although it is greater than that for children who have no family history of autoimmune disease. Nor is it always the same disease that runs in families. For example, a mother may have Graves' disease, while her daughter develops insulin-dependent diabetes mellitus.

● Could my thyroid condition explain why I did badly in my exams?

It is likely to be hyperthyroidism which affects people who are the right age to be taking exams. If it is not adequately treated, a reduced ability to concentrate will certainly lead to a substandard performance and the specialist will be happy to write to the relevant headteacher or college tutor to explain the problem.

● Could thyroid disease have caused my anxiety/depression?

The answer is almost certainly 'no', although hyperthyroidism and hypothyroidism will make underlying psychiatric illness worse. Unfortunately, even when a person with hyperthyroidism is successfully treated so that their overactive thyroid is brought under control, their psychiatric symptoms don't disappear altogether, although they may improve.

● Will my Graves' disease recur?

If your hyperthyroidism has been effectively treated with iodine-131, it will never return. If the hyperthyroidism has settled after a single course of carbimazole there is a 30 to 50 per cent chance of recurrence, usually within one to two years of stopping the drug. Recurrent hyperthyroidism after surgery is usually apparent within a few weeks but may occur as long as 40 years after apparently successful surgery.

● Does it matter if I forget to take my medication?

The occasional missed tablet is not the end of the world. Indeed symptoms of hypothyroidism due to lack of thyroxine are not usually felt for two to three weeks after stopping the tablets so it would still be possible to enjoy a seven to 10 day holiday if you'd inadvertently left your medication at home.

However, this is not to be recommended. Also patients with hypothyroidism may have other autoimmune diseases such as diabetes mellitus. Failure to take thyroxine regularly will affect the response to insulin and may lead to unexpected coma due to a low blood sugar.

Again, missing the odd carbimazole dose will not cause significant problems but symptoms of hyperthyroidism are likely to develop if you don't take the tablets for 24 to 48 hours, especially within a few weeks of starting treatment.

● I feel better when I am taking a higher dose of thyroxine than recommended by my doctor. Is this safe?

There is considerable debate about the correct dose of thyroxine. The consensus is that enough should be given to ensure that levels of T_4 in the blood are at the upper limit of normal or slightly elevated and TSH at the lower limit of normal, or in some patients undetectable. Although by taking excessive thyroxine a sense of well-being, increased energy and even weight loss may be achieved in the short term, there are long-term dangers to the heart and a possibility of increasing the rate of bone thinning and therefore encouraging the development of osteoporosis.

● Will tests involving radioactivity affect my fertility?

Definitely not. The amount of radioactivity involved is tiny – less than that in a X-ray so you have absolutely no cause for concern.

● Can treatment for Graves' disease make me fat?

No, although you will probably put back any weight you lost before your condition was diagnosed and treated.

However, there's no reason why you should end up weighing any more than you did before you started to develop Graves' disease.

● My daughter was put on thyroxine tablets at birth because she was hypothyroid. Will she have to take them forever?

Not necessarily. She will be taken off them then given a blood test when she's around a year to see whether she still needs them.

● **Is the time of day when I take my thyroxine tablets important?**

No, but most people find it's better to take them at the same time each day – that way you're less likely to forget.

Useful Addresses

The British Thyroid Foundation and Thyroid Eye Disease (TED) association, whose addresses are given below, are patient support groups.

British Thyroid Foundation

PO Box 97
Clifford, Wetherby
West Yorkshire LS23 6XD

The British Thyroid Foundation became a registered charity in 1991 and is run by volunteers who are committed to helping the thyroid disease sufferer. The principal aims of the Foundation are to provide support and clear information to sufferers of thyroid disorders, to promote a greater awareness of these disorders among the general public and the medical profession, to help to set up regional support groups and to raise funds for research.

Thyroid Eye Disease (TED)

71 Fore Street
Chudleigh
Devon
TQ13 0HT

Glossary

This glossary explains the meaning of the most frequently used clinical and related terms connected with the diagnosis and treatment of thyroid disorders.

carbimazole: the drug most commonly used in the UK in the treatment of hyperthyroidism. It acts by interfering with the excessive production of thyroid hormones.

de Quervain's thyroiditis: a form of viral thyroiditis that can occur following a viral infection of the thyroid.

exophthalmos: prominence of the eyes most commonly found in patients with hyperthyroidism caused by Graves' disease. The exophthalmos may affect one or both eyes, may be apparent before the overactive thyroid gland develops and may appear for the first time after successful treatment of the hyperthyroidism.

fine needle aspiration (FNA): a test that involves passing a small needle into the thyroid gland and sucking out (aspirating) a small sample of tissue for examination under the microscope. This technique often avoids the need for surgery in patients with certain types of goitre.

goitre: an enlarged thyroid gland.

Graves' disease: the name given to the most common form of hyperthyroidism. Patients often have exophthalmos, a goitre and sometimes raised red patches on the legs known as pretibial myxoedema.

Hashimoto's thyroiditis: the name given to a particular kind of goitre caused by autoimmune disease. Although the thyroid gland is enlarged, there is often evidence of hypothyroidism.

hyperthyroidism: condition resulting from an overactive thyroid gland.

hypothyroidism: condition resulting from an underactive thyroid gland.

myxoedema: this means the same as hypothyroidism, but is often used to describe patients in whom the thyroid underactivity is severe and of long standing.

postpartum thyroiditis: a transient disturbance in the balance of the thyroid gland which can occur in the first year after childbirth. There are usually no symptoms, but there may be symptoms of hyperthyroidism or hypothyroidism. Treatment is not usually necessary.

propranolol (Inderal): a drug belonging to the group known as beta-blockers which alleviate some of the symptoms, e.g. tremor in patients with an overactive thyroid gland. Other members of the group include nadolol (Corgard) and sotalol (Sotacor).

proptosis: another word for exophthalmos.

propylthiouracil: this drug has a similar action to carbimazole. It is used if patients develop side effects to carbimazole and is increasingly prescribed to patients who are pregnant or breastfeeding when hyperthyroid.

radioactive iodine (iodine-131): an isotope of iodine which is used on the investigation and treatment of hyperthyroidism.

thyroglobulin: a protein secreted by the thyroid gland. Its measurement is an important part of the follow-up of patients who have been treated for thyroid cancer. It is known as a 'tumour marker' because its presence in certain situations may indicate that the cancer has returned to other parts of the body.

triiodothyronine (T_3): a hormone which, along with thyroxine, is secreted by the thyroid gland. It is responsible for controlling the metabolism of the body. Although available in tablet form, it is not usually prescribed for patients with hypothyroidism because it does not provide such good control as thyroxine.

thyrotoxicosis: another term for hyperthyroidism.

thyroxine (T_4): a hormone secreted, along with triiodothyronine, by the thyroid gland. It has to be converted in the body to triiodothyronine before it is active. Thyroxine is available in tablet form for the treatment of hypothyroidism.

thyrotrophin (thyroid-stimulating hormone, TSH): a hormone secreted by the pituitary gland and responsible for controlling the output of thyroid hormones by the thyroid gland. In hypothyroidism caused by disease of the thyroid gland, TSH concentrations are elevated in the blood and in hyperthyroidism TSH concentrations are low.

Index

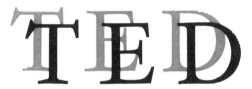

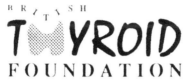